T0383936

iUniverse books may be ordered through booksellers or by contacting:

iUniverse
1663 Liberty Drive
Bloomington, IN 47403
www.iuniverse.com
844-349-9409

Because of the dynamic nature of the Internet, any web addresses or links contained in this book may have changed since publication and may no longer be valid. The views expressed in this work are solely those of the author and do not necessarily reflect the views of the publisher, and the publisher hereby disclaims any responsibility for them.

Any people depicted in stock imagery provided by Getty Images are models, and such images are being used for illustrative purposes only. Certain stock imagery © Getty Images.

ISBN: 978-1-6632-5587-7 (sc)
ISBN: 978-1-6632-5588-4 (e)

Print information available on the last page.

iUniverse rev. date: 10/25/2024

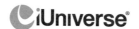

Understanding Food Allergies

A GUIDE FOR KIDS

SARA COMITO

Dear Reader,

Chances are, if you are reading this book, you may have food allergies or someone you know is affected by them. At first, allergies may seem very scary, confusing and may even make you feel different, but I wrote this book for you to realize that it is a common problem for many kids just like you.

You see, even if you are the one with the allergy, it affects everyone around you. My little brother Massimo and my little sister Eva both are affected by severe allergies. I live every day being aware of what allergens are in foods that may affect them. From a very early age, Massimo was diagnosed with 27 food allergies resulting in reactions from skin rashes to violent vomiting. As a 4 year old, I was terrified to see him go through one of his reactions. Slowly but surely, we managed to figure out how to deal with them and comfort him.

The aim of this book, is to educate you about the most common food allergies, understand why your body reacts the way it does and how to hopefully avoid and/or manage allergic reactions.

Your friend,
Sara

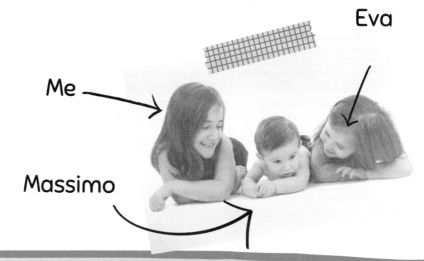

Eva

Me

Massimo

Table of Contents

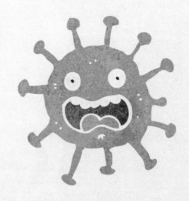

What are Food Allergies

Allergens   P. 3
Antibodies   P. 4-5
Allergic reactions   P. 6-8

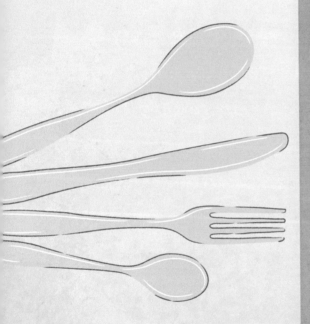

10 Most Common Allergens

Peanuts   P. 11
Tree nuts   P.12
Milk   P.13-14
Eggs   P. 15
Mustard   P. 16
Crustaceans & Molluscs   P. 17
Fish   P. 18
Sesame   P. 19
Soy   P. 20
Wheat & Triticale   P. 21-22

Living with Food Allergies

Prevention   P. 25-26
Cross-contamination   P. 27-28

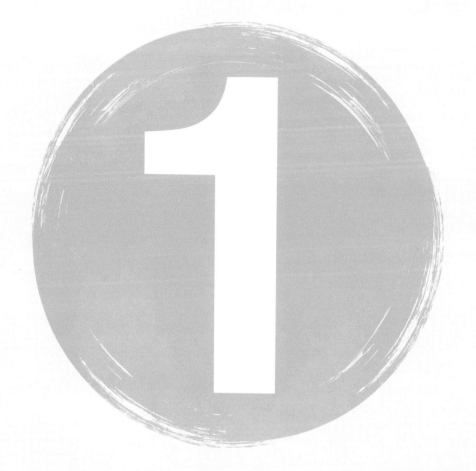

WHAT ARE FOOD ALLERGIES?

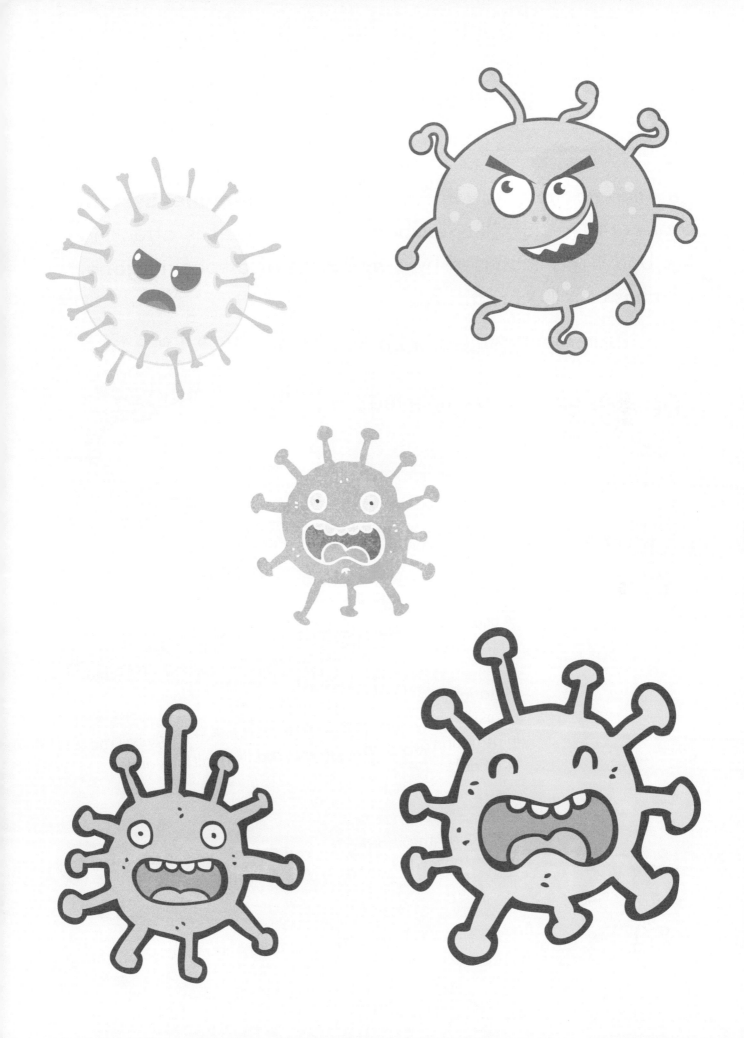

Allergens

An allergic reaction occurs when the **immune system** overreacts to an **allergen** because it thinks it is attacking the body. This is caused by a **mutation** of a specific **gene,** which is usually **hereditary**.

Allergens can either be airborne:
pollen, animal hair, etc.

or They can also be ingested :
food or a substance in food.

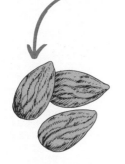

Immune system :
The system in the body that helps fight infections and diseases.

Allergen :
A usually harmless substance that can trigger a response in the immune system and can lead to an allergic reaction.

Mutation :
A mistake or a change in DNA (material that carries all the information about how a living organism will look and function).

Gene :
Genes carry the information that determines the features that are passed onto you by your parents.

Hereditary :
The passing on of characteristics from parents to kids.

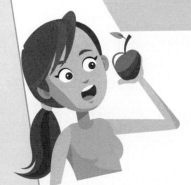

Protein:
A large biological molecule. There are many different types and are very essential to living beings.

The reaction caused by the allergen triggers the release of antibodies. The antibodies are the cause of the genetic mutation. They are Y shaped **proteins** that neutralize components from outside of the body.

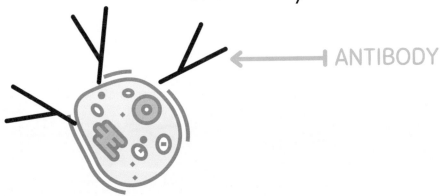

ANTIBODY

They are shaped to attach to a specific type of allergen. Just like a **LOCK AND KEY**. An antibody can only recognize one allergen. This is why a person can be allergic to peanuts and not to eggs.

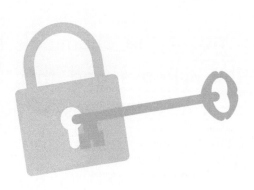

4

Antibodies

The **antibodies** will travel and attach to specialized **cells** in your body that act like security guards. The cells are found on the skin, nose and mucus membranes. The cells create chemicals to flush out the **allergen**. The chemicals and their effects are what causes an allergic reaction.

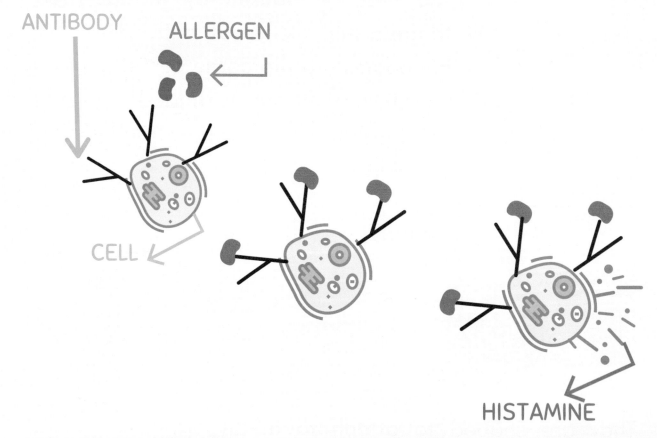

ANTIBODY

ALLERGEN

CELL

HISTAMINE

One of the chemicals is called **histamine**. Histamine closes the airways and thus making it difficult to breath. It also expands the vessels which causes fluid leakage. Another chemical is called leukotrienes and it causes excessive mucus that results in a runny nose.

The chemicals produced by the cells cause several different reactions. Here are the main reactions:

Watery eyes

Stomache ache

Difficulty breathing, coughing

Hives or rashes

Runny nose

Vomiting

Allergic Reactions

Anaphylaxis is a life threatening allergic reaction that affects the whole body. This reaction can make it difficult to breath, drop blood pressure and affect heart rate. It can happen within seconds, minutes or hours after ingesting the food containing the allergen. Possible symptoms may vary for each person.

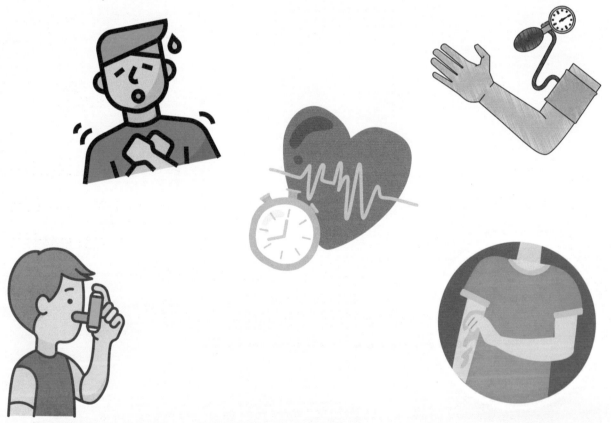

It has been proven that there is a direct link between eczema, asthma and allergies because they share the same gene. Chances are, if you suffer from one of the above, you may also experience the others.

EPIPEN

When an allergic reaction occurs, it is important to act QUICKLY (especially if it is an anaphylaxis reaction) and take a dose of epinephrine (adrenaline), also known as the EpiPen. Make sure to read the instructions beforehand. Here's a little trick to help you remember what to do :

BLUE TO THE SKY
ORANGE TO THE THIGH

Epinephrine relaxes the muscles of the airways to help the person breathe and increases the person's heart rate which helps improve the blood flow. It is important for people with allergies to ALWAYS carry an EpiPen with them. It is also important to have 2 doses available in case of a secondary reaction.

After taking a dose of epinephrine, it is important to call 911 and head straight to the hospital because there may be side effets to taking the EpiPen. Possible side effects include anxiety, restlessness, dizziness and shakiness.

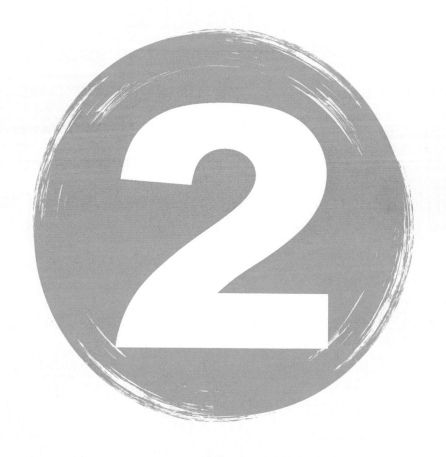

10 MOST COMMON ALLERGENS

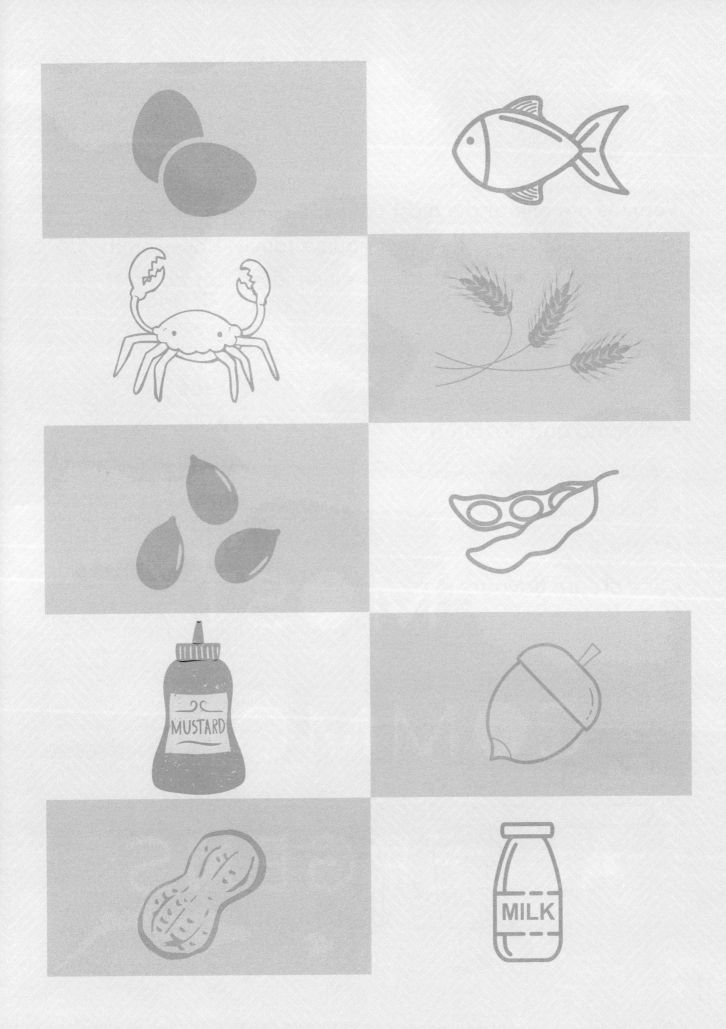

Peanuts

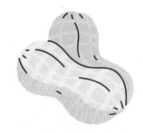

Peanuts are one of the most common allergies affecting children. They are part of the legume family. However, it is important to note that they are unrelated to tree nuts.

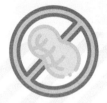 Beware of peanuts in the following products:

- Almond and Hazelnut paste
- Baked goods
- Cereal
- Ice cream flavours
- Peanut oil
- Peanut butter

- Asian cuisine
- Candies
- Granola
- Salad dressings & toppings
- Trail mix

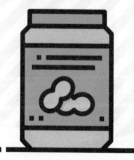

Lupin is a legume that belongs to the same plant family as peanuts and some people are allergic to both. It is recommended for people who are allergic to peanuts to also avoid lupins.

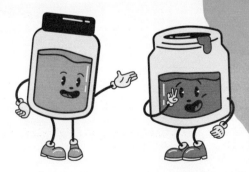

There are several different types of tree nuts. If you are allergic to one tree nut, it is very probable that you are also allergic to some of the other ones too.

Here is a list of the most common tree nuts:

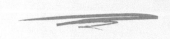

Tree nuts can be found in:

Almonds

Cashews

Chestnuts

Hazelnuts

Pistachios

Pecans

Walnuts

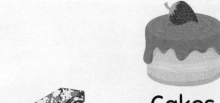

Cakes

Chocolate

Ice Cream

Granola Bars

Pies

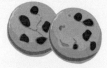

Cookies

Milk

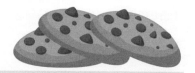

A milk allergy is caused by a reaction to the protein in cow's milk. This is an allergy that is commonly outgrown. There are many other substitutes to cow's milk such as, soy, almond, oat, coconut and cashew to name a few. Be aware that milk could also be found in several baked goods, cereal, cookies, milk chocolate, etc.

Lactose:
A sugar present in milk, therefore it is also present in other dairy products such as yogurt, butter and cheese.

Molecules:
A group of atoms linked together by chemical bonds.

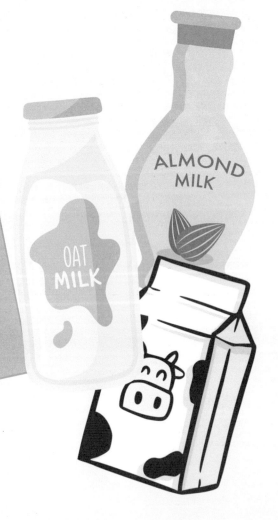

LACTOSE INTOLERANCE

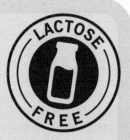

A milk allergy is very different from lactose intolerance. An intolerance is when the body cannot digest any product that contains lactose. Digestion is when your body cuts molecules of food into little pieces so it could travel from our intestines into our blood. In order for this to happen our body needs a protein called enzymes.

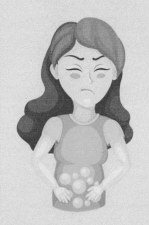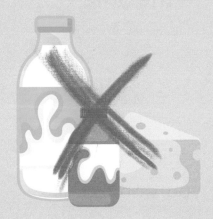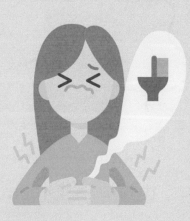

If there is an absence of enzymes, problems may occur during digestion. Instead of the food getting digested, it accumulates which creates unwanted symptoms such as bloating and diarrhea. A good alternative to cow's milk is soy milk as it doesn't contain lactose.

Eggs

An egg allergy is most common in young children and can be outgrown within a few years.

The egg has two allergenic parts, the **yolk** and the **white**.

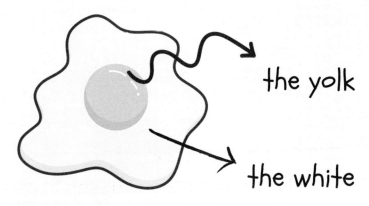

the yolk

the white

Even though you are allergic to eggs, it is possible that you can eat eggs as long as they are well cooked.

For example, in a birthday cake.

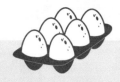

Eggs are used in many different foods. Here are some possible sources where eggs can be found:

Drinks

Baby food

Desserts

Candy

Icing

Pasta

Soups

Sauces

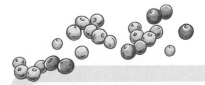

Mustard comes from a plant that is part of the Brassicaceae family. In this case, it is the mustard **seed** that is the allergen.

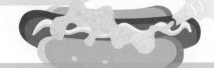

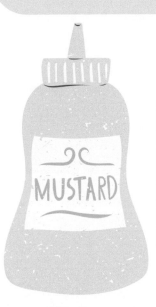

Possible sources where this allergen can be found is in salad dressings and sauces. Mustard is also used in many cuisines, including Indian, Italian, Eastern European and Middle Eastern dishes.

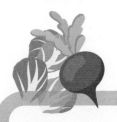

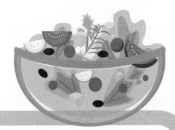

The Brassicaceae family includes broccoli, canola, cauliflower, cabbage, brussel sprouts and turnips. People with a mustard allergy should avoid consuming the seeds from the other members of the Brassicaceae family because they can possibly also cause a reaction.

Crustaceans & Molluscs

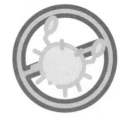

Crustaceans and Molluscs are aquatic animals otherwise known as **shellfish**. This allergen isn't very common in children. It mostly affects adults. It is an allergen that is usually present throughout their entire life.

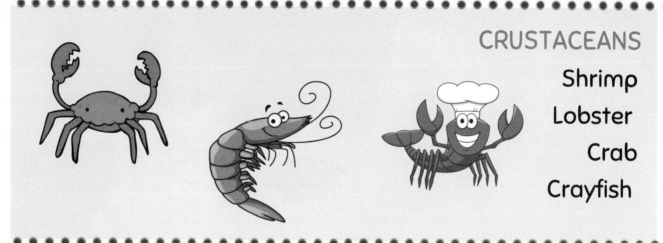

CRUSTACEANS

Shrimp
Lobster
Crab
Crayfish

MOLLUSCS

Clams

Mussels

Octopus

Oysters

Scallops

Snails

Squid

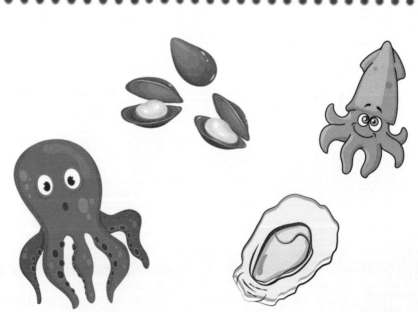

Crustaceans and Molluscs can also be found in sushi and sashimi.

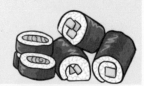

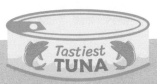

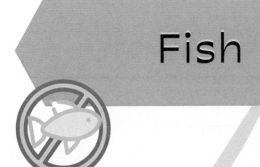

Just like the crustacean and molluscs allergen, a fish allergy is more common in adults and is usually lifelong.

Some people can experience a reaction from exposure to the strong cooking smell.

There are hundreds of different types of fish. Some of the most common ones are salmon, swordfish, trout, sardines and tuna.

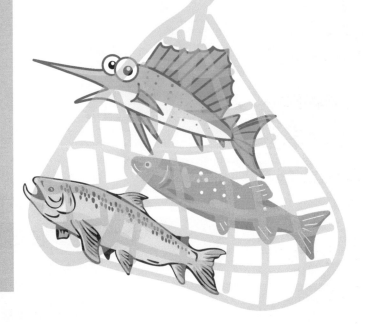

Sesame

Sesame is a flowering plant that produces edible seeds. Tahini is the name of the paste made from sesame seeds.

Sesame can be found in:

SESAME SALT

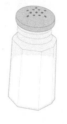

BREADS

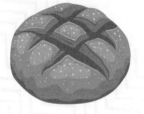

BAGELS

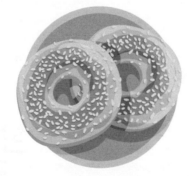

SESAME OIL

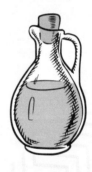

VEGETABLE OIL
(MAY CONTAIN)

HUMMUS

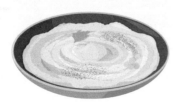

HAMBURGER BUNS

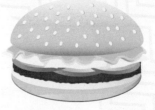

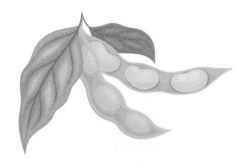

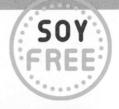

SOY FREE

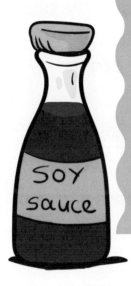

Soy comes from soybeans and is a type of legume. Soybeans can be made into flour, milk, tofu, oil, etc.

A soy allergy is most common in children and it can be outgrown.

Soy can be found in salad dressings, snack foods, miso soup, baby formula, breaded foods, etc.

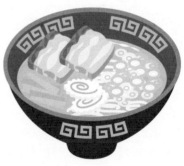

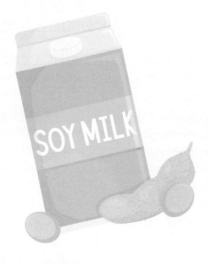

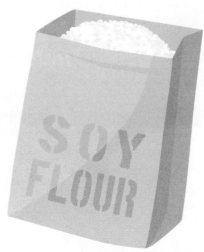

20

Wheat & Triticale

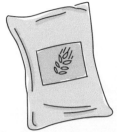

Triticale is a grain containing a mix of both wheat and rye. A wheat allergy usually developpes in children and it can be outgrown. However, adults who develop the allergy are most likely to have it for life.

Wheat allergy and **celiac disease** are two different conditions. A wheat allergy is when the immune system reacts badly to a protein found in wheat. See the next page for more explanation on what celiac disease is.

Wheat and triticale are the main ingredients found in baked goods such as bread, breadcrumbs, cakes, cereal, cookies, crackers, donuts, muffins, batter-fried foods, and chocolate.

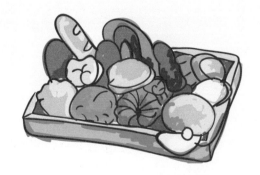

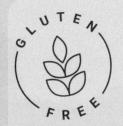

CELIAC DISEASE

When a person suffering from Celiac Disease ingests food containing the protein gluten (found in wheat, rye and barley), an immune system reaction happens. It then causes damage to the small intestine and stops the body from absorbing nutrients.

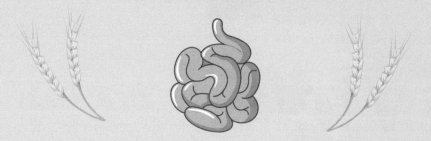

This can lead to anemia, diarrhea, weight loss, fatigue, stomach cramps and bloating.

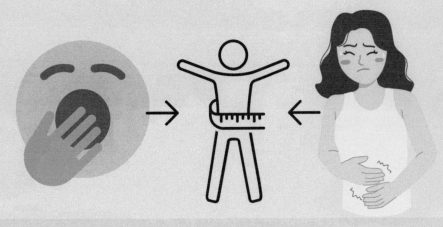

LIVING WITH FOOD ALLERGIES

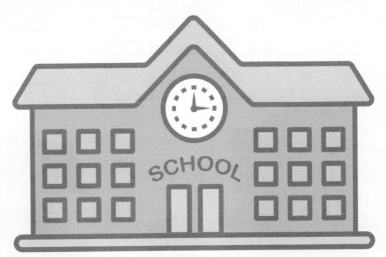

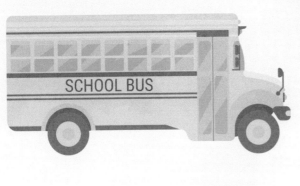

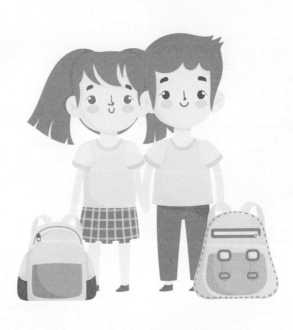

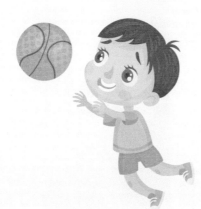

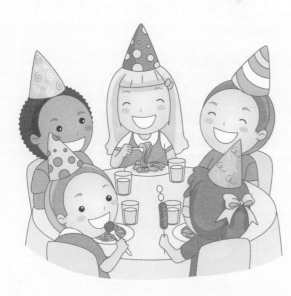

Prevention

Food allergies can be present in foods you wouldn't expect. That is why it is necessary to **ALWAYS** check the labels and read the ingredients list.

> ## IT IS SUGGESTED TO TRIPLE CHECK WHEN READING LABELS.

Nutrition Facts

Serving Size oz.
Serving Per Container

Amount Per Serving:

Calories	Calories From Fat

	% Daily value*
Total Fat	%
Saturated Fat	%
Trans Fat	
Cholesterol	%
Sodium	%
Total Carbohydrate	%
Dietary Fiber	%
Sugars	
Protein	

*Percent Daily values are based on a 2000 calorie diet. Your daily values may be higher or lewer depending on you calorie needs.

Read once at the store before purchasing.

Read again when you get home before putting it away.

And, one last time before eating the product.

When eating out, it is important to be **prepared**. If eating at a friend's house, advise the host about your allergies. You can also bring your own meal to avoid any inconvenience to the host. Bringing your own dessert at a birthday party also avoids any feelings about missing out!

If going out to eat at a restaurant, be sure to research the restaurant's menu online before going. Advise the waiter about your allergies. **Don't forget** to inquire about cross-contamination. It is strongly suggested to always have **2** EpiPens with you at all times.

DON'T FORGET!

BLUE TO THE SKY,

ORANGE TO THE THIGH.

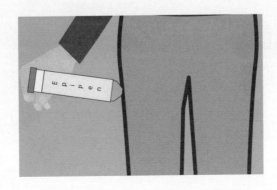

Cross - Contamination

Cross-contamination can happen when a small amount of a food allergen accidentally comes into contact with another food. There are **3** possible ways that cross-contamination could happen.

1 FOOD TO FOOD :

An example of food to food cross-contamination is picking almonds out of a salad. Even though the almonds are not physically in the salad anymore, it has contaminated the salad with its residue.

2 FOOD TO OBJECT :

An example of food to object is when someone uses a knife to cut salmon and uses that same knife, without washing it, to cut meat. The salmon allergen gets transferred onto the meat because the knife wasn't washed.

3 FOOD TO SALIVA :

An example of food transmitted by saliva is when two people kiss and one of them ate something the other person is allergic to.

Cross - Contamination

Don't share food, utensils, napkins or drinks !

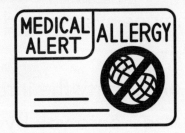

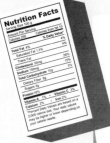

Read ingredient labels !

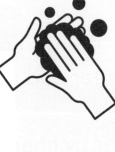

Wash hands before and after eating !

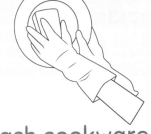

Wash cookware like pots and pans !

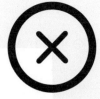

Don't buy items that say "may contain" !

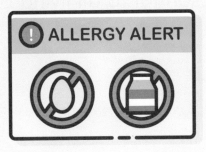

GLOSSARY :

Allergen :

A usually harmless substance that can trigger a response in the immune system and can lead to an allergic reaction.

Gene :

Genes carry the information that determines the traits that are passed onto you by your parents.

Hereditary :

The passing on of characteristics from parents to kids.

Immune system :

The system in the body that helps fight infections and diseases.

Lactose :

A sugar present in milk, therefore it is also present in other dairy products such as yogurt, butter and cheese.

Molecules :

A group of atomes linked together by chemical bonds.

Mutation :

A mistake or a change in DNA (material that carries all the information about how a living organism will look and function).

Protein :

A large biological molecule. There are many types and they are essential to all living beings.

BIBLIOGRAPHY :

Magazine:

Demizieux, Laurent. "Allergies Et Intolérances Alimentaires." Cosinus, Le Magazine De Maths Et De Scienceno. n°188, December 2016.

Websites:

"Food Allergies: Causes, Symptoms & Treatment." ACAAI Public Website, November 7, 2022. https://acaai.org/allergies/types/food-allergy.

"Allergies: A Scientific Explanation." Dartmouth Undergraduate Journal of Science. Accessed March 21, 2023. https://sites.dartmouth.edu/dujs/2015/03/12/allergies-a-scientific-explanation/.

"Food Allergy & Anaphylaxis: Psychological Impacts: Psychological Impacts." Food Allergy & Anaphylaxis | Psychological Impacts | Psychological Impacts. Accessed March 21, 2023. https://www.foodallergyawareness.org/food-allergy-and-anaphylaxis/psychological-impacts/psychological-impacts/.

"Allergies Archive." Food Allergy Canada. Accessed March 21, 2023. https://foodallergycanada.ca/allergies/.

ICONOGRAPHY :

Page 2:

Siblings. 2009. Photograph.

Printed in the United States
by Baker & Taylor Publisher Services